Easy Low Histamine Diet Cookbook

The Ultimate Quick And Easy Delicious Recipes For Histamine Intolerance Management

Rose V Allen

Copyright © [2023] Rose V. Allen

All rights reserved. No part of this book may be reproduced in any form or by any electronic or mechanical means, including information storage and retrieval systems, without permission in writing from the author, except by a reviewer who may quote brief passages in a review.

This book is not intended to replace professional advice from a qualified professional. The author recommends seeking the advice of a qualified professional before taking any action based on the information contained in this book.

ABOUT THE AUTHOR

Rose V. Allen is a passionate nutritionist based in the United States, dedicated to helping individuals optimize their health and well-being through evidence-based dietary strategies. With a deep-rooted belief in the transformative power of food, Rose has spent years honing her expertise in the field of nutrition, specializing in the management of histamine intolerance.

Armed with a Bachelor's degree in Nutrition Science from a prestigious institution, Rose has acquired a comprehensive understanding of the intricate relationship between diet and health. Her journey in the field of nutrition has been marked by a relentless pursuit of knowledge, fueled by a genuine desire to empower others to take control of their health and vitality.

Drawing on her extensive experience working with clients from diverse backgrounds, Rose has developed a unique approach to managing histamine intolerance that emphasizes practicality, flavor, and flexibility. Through her personalized counseling sessions, workshops, and educational resources, she has helped countless individuals navigate the complexities of histamine intolerance with confidence and ease.

As the author of the "Easy Low Histamine Diet Cookbook," Rose brings her wealth of knowledge and expertise to the forefront, providing readers with a comprehensive guide to managing histamine intolerance through diet. With a focus on simplicity, accessibility, and deliciousness, Rose's recipes offer a welcome respite from the restrictive nature of traditional low-histamine diets, proving that eating well can be both enjoyable and nourishing.

Outside of her work as a nutritionist and author, Rose is a dedicated advocate for holistic health and wellness. She believes in the power of community and collaboration to effect positive change, and she actively engages with her audience through social media, workshops, and speaking engagements.

Driven by her passion for helping others lead healthier, happier lives, Rose continues to inspire and empower individuals to embrace a mindful approach to eating, one delicious bite at a time.

TABLE OF CONTENT

INTRODUCTION

Histamine intolerance is more than simply a dietary limitation; it's a daily struggle against pain, uncertainty, and the ongoing desire for balance. The symptoms — ranging from headaches and stomach disorders to skin rashes and respiratory problems – may be severe, influencing every part of life, from what you eat to how you mingle and travel.

It's a syndrome that frequently leaves persons feeling alienated, dissatisfied, and overwhelmed by the constraints put on their lives.

But within these problems lies an opportunity – a chance to regain control over your health and well-being, to embrace a new way of eating that not only alleviates symptoms but also enables you to flourish.

This cookbook is your passport to that journey, delivering a treasure trove of fast, simple, and tasty dishes that cater to the requirements of persons with histamine intolerance.

Gone are the days of drab, uninspired dinners and lengthy hours spent exploring grocery store aisles for safe choices. In these pages, you'll find a world of culinary pleasures that show you don't have to trade flavor for health. From substantial breakfasts to full dinners and decadent sweets, each meal is precisely prepared to excite your taste buds while sticking to low histamine principles.

But this cookbook is more than simply a compilation of recipes - it's a lifeline, a light of hope for people navigating the tumultuous seas of histamine intolerance.

It's a tribute to the endurance of the human spirit and the power of community, bringing together people from all walks of life who share a similar objective - to recover their health and vitality.

So, whether you're a seasoned chef or a newbie in the kitchen, whether you're going on this road alone or with the support of loved ones by your side, know that you are not alone. Within these pages, you'll discover not only nutrition for your body but also consolation for your spirit, as you start on a transforming path towards improved health and well-being.

Together, we'll manage the hurdles, celebrate the wins, and appreciate every delicious mouthful along the road. Welcome to the "Easy Low Histamine Diet Cookbook" — where relief, sustenance, and culinary joy greet you at every step.

Let's go on this adventure together and find the pleasure of eating properly, living completely, and flourishing despite histamine intolerance.

Hypersensitivity to Histamine: A Synopsis

An impaired capacity to metabolize histamine—a chemical that plays a role in immunological reactions, digestion, and neurological system function—defines histamine intolerance. The enzymes diamine oxidase (DAO) and histamine N-methyltransferase (HNMT) normally break down histamine. Those who are histamine intolerant, on the other hand, may have an overabundance of histamine because these enzymes are either underactive or overworked.

Histamine intolerance symptoms may range from mild to severe and can manifest in a variety of ways. Some people have headaches, migraines, vertigo, flushing, congestion in the nose, gastrointestinal problems (including bloating, diarrhea, and stomach discomfort), skin rashes, and even anxiety and panic episodes. It is possible to induce these symptoms by eating foods that are high in histamine or that either inhibit DAO action or enhance histamine release.

The Value of Nutritional Counselling

To control symptoms of histamine intolerance, dietary management is essential. Because histamine is found naturally in a wide variety of foods, those who are histamine intolerant may greatly benefit from knowing which foods to restrict or avoid to reduce their symptoms and enhance their quality of life.

A low-histamine diet may help with this, since it encourages reducing consumption of foods high in histamine while also taking processing, storage, and freshness into account, among other things.

By carefully choosing meals and implementing dietary adjustments, persons with histamine intolerance may decrease their exposure to histamine and other histamine-releasing chemicals, therefore minimizing the frequency and severity of symptoms.

Additionally, treating any underlying gastrointestinal disorders and supporting the body's natural histamine-clearing systems will further boost the efficiency of dietary control.

How This Cookbook Can Help

This cookbook is particularly developed to enable those with histamine intolerance to efficiently control their illness via food. It presents a broad choice of tasty and healthy meals that conform to the principles of a low-histamine diet while yet delivering diversity and taste. Here's how this cookbook can help:

Recipe range: The cookbook contains a varied range of dishes spanning numerous cultures and meal kinds, ensuring that those with histamine intolerance have plenty of alternatives to pick from. Each dish is meticulously developed to be low in histamine and free from typical trigger items, making meal planning and preparation quicker and more pleasurable.

Ingredient Substitutions: For persons with histamine sensitivity, specific substances may need to be swapped to lower histamine levels or prevent triggering symptoms. This cookbook gives useful hints and recommendations for ingredient replacements, enabling users to personalize recipes according to their dietary requirements and tastes without compromising flavor or nutritional value.

Nutritional advice: In addition to giving tasty recipes, this cookbook also gives vital nutritional advice and information to assist those with histamine intolerance make educated decisions about their diet. It offers recommendations on meal planning, grocery shopping, and food preparation, as well as advice on combining nutrient-rich items that promote general health and well-being.

Education and Empowerment: By providing persons with histamine intolerance with practical skills and resources, this cookbook enables them to take charge of their diet and manage their illness more successfully. It provides a feeling of strength and independence, enabling people to enjoy meals without worry of causing unpleasant symptoms.

CHAPTER ONE

Understanding Histamine Intolerance

What is Histamine Intolerance?

An impaired capacity to metabolize histamine—a chemical that plays a role in immunological reactions, digestion, and neurological system function—defines histamine intolerance. Histamine is naturally created by the body and is also contained in some foods. In healthy persons, histamine is broken down by enzymes including diamine oxidase (DAO) and histamine N-methyltransferase (HNMT). However, in persons with histamine intolerance, these enzymes may be insufficient or overloaded, leading to a buildup of histamine in the body.

Common Symptoms and Triggers

Symptoms of histamine intolerance may vary considerably and may impact numerous systems in the body. Some typical symptoms include:

- **Gastrointestinal Issues:** These may include stomach discomfort, bloating, diarrhea, constipation, nausea, and vomiting.

- **Skin Reactions:** Histamine intolerance might appear as skin rashes, itching, hives, eczema, or flushing.

- **Respiratory Symptoms:** Nasal congestion, sneezing, runny nose, coughing, and trouble breathing may develop.

- **Neurological Symptoms:** Headaches, migraines, dizziness, exhaustion, sleeplessness, and cognitive impairment are prevalent.

- **Cardiovascular Symptoms:** Rapid heartbeat, palpitations, and low blood pressure may develop in certain circumstances.

Common causes for histamine intolerance include:

Histamine-Rich Foods: Foods rich in histamine content include aged cheeses, fermented foods (such as sauerkraut and kimchi), cured meats, smoked fish, and alcoholic drinks (particularly wine and beer).

Histamine-Releasing Meals: Some meals may induce the release of histamine in the body, even if they are not fundamentally rich in histamine. These include citrus fruits, tomatoes, strawberries, spinach, and chocolate.

DAO-Inhibiting Foods: Certain foods include substances that impede the function of diamine oxidase (DAO), the enzyme responsible for breaking down histamine in the stomach. Examples include alcohol, black tea, green tea, energy drinks, and certain pharmaceuticals.

Food Additives and Preservatives: Some additives and preservatives, such as sulfites, benzoates, and nitrites, may also induce histamine release or interfere with DAO action.

Diagnostic Process and Testing

Diagnosing histamine intolerance may be hard since it combines symptoms with other illnesses, such as food allergies, irritable bowel syndrome (IBS), and mast cell activation syndrome (MCAS). The diagnostic method often involves:

Medical History: Your healthcare professional will question your symptoms, medical history, and dietary habits to examine the probability of histamine intolerance.

Elimination Diet: A low-histamine diet may be prescribed to evaluate whether symptoms improve with decreased histamine consumption. This entails avoiding histamine-rich meals and other possible triggers for some time.

Food journal: Keeping a comprehensive food journal may help monitor symptoms and identify possible trigger foods or patterns of symptom worsening.

Laboratory Tests: Blood tests to evaluate DAO levels or histamine levels may be conducted, however, their reliability and accuracy are still contested within the medical profession.

Response to Treatment: If symptoms improve with dietary adjustments or drugs that lower histamine levels, it may support a diagnosis of histamine intolerance.

CHAPTER TWO

The Basics of a Low Histamine Diet

Principles of Low Histamine Eating

A low histamine diet is meant to decrease the consumption of histamine-rich foods and other items that might stimulate histamine release or impede the function of diamine oxidase (DAO), the enzyme that's in charge of breaking down histamine in the gut. The fundamental elements of a reduced histamine diet include:

Avoiding rich Histamine Foods: This includes foods that are naturally rich in histamine or have been aged, fermented, or processed in a manner that raises histamine levels. Examples include aged cheeses, fermented meals (such as sauerkraut and yogurt), cured meats, smoked fish, and alcoholic drinks.

Limiting Histamine-Releasing Meals: Some meals may induce the release of histamine in the body, even if they are not fundamentally rich in histamine. These include citrus fruits, tomatoes, strawberries, spinach, and chocolate. While these meals don't need to be fully removed, it's advised to take them in moderation.

Avoiding DAO-Inhibiting Foods: Certain foods include substances that may hinder the action of diamine oxidase (DAO), the enzyme responsible for breaking down histamine in the stomach. Examples include alcohol, black tea, green tea, energy drinks, and certain pharmaceuticals. Minimizing the intake of certain items may assist promote histamine metabolism.

Foods to Include and Avoid

Foods to Include:

Fresh Meats and Poultry: Freshly cooked meats and poultry are often low in histamine compared to processed or cured meats. Opt for fresh cuts and avoid processed or aged meats.

Fresh Fish and shellfish: newly caught or newly frozen fish and shellfish are often lower in histamine compared to smoked or canned kinds. Choose fresh fish and seafood whenever feasible.

Fresh Fruits and Vegetables: Most fresh fruits and vegetables are well-tolerated on a low histamine diet. However, certain people may need to avoid high-histamine foods like citrus fruits, tomatoes, and strawberries, depending on their tolerance levels.

Gluten-Free Grains: Grains including rice, quinoa, millet, and gluten-free oats are ideal for a low histamine diet. However, persons with gluten intolerance or sensitivity should ensure they purchase certified gluten-free items.

Fresh Dairy Alternatives: For individuals who accept dairy alternatives, such as rice milk, almond milk, or coconut milk, these may be used instead of dairy products. However, be careful with store-bought kinds, since some may include chemicals or preservatives that might exacerbate symptoms.

Foods to Avoid:

Aged Cheeses: Avoid aged cheeses such as cheddar, Parmesan, and blue cheese, which have greater histamine levels compared to fresh cheeses.

Fermented Foods: Steer clear of fermented foods like sauerkraut, kimchi, kombucha, and miso, since they are strong in histamine.

Cured and Processed Meats: Deli meats, bacon, sausage, and other cured or processed meats should be avoided owing to their high histamine level.

Smoked and Canned Fish: Smoked or canned fish, such as smoked salmon or canned tuna, should be avoided owing to their higher histamine levels.

Alcoholic Beverages: Alcohol, especially wine, beer, and champagne, should be reduced or avoided, since they might elevate histamine levels and impede DAO function.

CHAPTER THREE

Quick and Easy Breakfasts Recipe

Blueberry Banana Smoothie

This refreshing smoothie mixes the sweetness of blueberries and bananas with the earthy taste of spinach, providing a healthful and delightful morning choice.

Preparation Time: 5 minutes

Cooking Time: None

Total Time: 5 minutes

Serving Size: 1

Ingredients:

- 1 ripe banana, frozen
- 1/2 cup frozen blueberries
- 1/2 cup spinach leaves
- 1/2 cup Greek yogurt or dairy-free yogurt substitute
- 1 tablespoon nut butter (optional)

- 1/2 cup naturally almond milk or other milk that you prefer

Method of Preparation:

1. Place all items in a blender.
2. Blend until smooth and creamy.
3. Pour into a glass and drink immediately.

Quinoa Breakfast Bowl

This protein-packed breakfast dish has fluffy quinoa topped with creamy avocado, juicy tomato, and a flawlessly poached egg, delivering a delightful and healthy start to your day.

Preparation Time: 5 minutes

Cooking Time: 15 minutes (for quinoa and poached egg)

Total Time: 20 minutes

Serving Size: 1

Ingredients:

- 1/2 cup cooked quinoa

- 1/2 avocado, sliced

- 1/2 cup cherry tomatoes, halved

- 1 poached egg

- Salt & pepper, to taste

Method of Preparation:

1. Cook quinoa according to package directions.

2. Transfer cooked quinoa to a bowl.

3. Top with sliced avocado and cherry tomatoes.

4. Carefully add the poached egg on top.

5. Season with salt and pepper.

6. Serve immediately and enjoy!

Chia Seed Pudding

This creamy chia seed pudding is a make-ahead breakfast alternative that's filled with fiber and omega-3 fatty acids. Customize it with your favorite toppings for a delightful and healthy morning treat.

Preparation Time: 5 minutes (including overnight soaking)

Total Time: Overnight soaking + 5 minutes

Serving Size: 1

Ingredients:

- 1/4 cup chia seeds
- 1 cup unsweetened almond milk or other milk of choice
- 1/2 teaspoon vanilla extract
- Optional toppings: fresh berries, sliced banana, chopped almonds, shredded coconut, honey or maple syrup

Method of Preparation:

1. In a dish or container, mix chia seeds, almond milk, and vanilla essence.

2. Cover and refrigerate overnight, or for at least 4 hours, to let the chia seeds absorb the liquid and thicken.

3. Stir thoroughly before serving and add your favorite toppings, such as fresh berries, sliced banana, chopped almonds, shredded coconut, or a drizzle of honey or maple syrup.

4. Enjoy cold or at room temperature.

Egg Muffins

These delicious egg muffins are excellent for meal prep and on-the-go meals. Packed with protein and vegetables, they're a pleasant and healthy way to start your day.

Preparation Time: 10 minutes

Cooking Time: 20 minutes

Total Time: 30 minutes

Serving Size: 6 muffins

Ingredients:

- 6 eggs
- 1/4 cup milk or dairy-free milk substitute
- 1 cup diced veggies (such as bell peppers, spinach, onions, mushrooms)
- 1/2 cup shredded cheese (optional)
- Salt & pepper, to taste

Method of Preparation:

1. Preheat your oven to 350°F (175°C). Oil a muffin tray or prepare the muffin liners.

2. In a bowl, mix eggs and milk. Season with salt and pepper.

3. Stir in chopped veggies and shredded cheese, if using.

4. Divide the egg mixture equally among the muffin cups.

5. Bake for 20-25 minutes, or until the egg muffins are firm and golden brown on top.

6. Allow to cool slightly before removing from the muffin tray.

7. Serve warm or keep in an airtight jar in the refrigerator for up to 5 days.

Coconut Flour Pancakes

These fluffy coconut flour pancakes are gluten-free and low in histamine, making them a fantastic alternative for individuals with dietary requirements. Enjoy them topped with fresh fruit and a sprinkle of honey or maple syrup for a delightful morning treat.

Preparation Time: 10 minutes

Cooking Time: 10 minutes

Total Time: 20 minutes

Serving Size: 2-3 pancakes

Ingredients:

- 1/4 cup coconut flour
- 2 eggs
- 1/4 cup natural almond milk or other milk that you like
- 1 tablespoon coconut oil, melted
- 1/2 teaspoon baking powder

- 1/2 teaspoon vanilla extract

- Pinch of salt

Method of Preparation

1. In a bowl, mix eggs, almond milk, melted coconut oil, and vanilla extract.

2. In a separate dish, whisk together coconut flour, baking powder, and salt.

3. Gradually add the dry ingredients to the wet components, stirring until fully blended and no lumps remain.

4. Allow the batter to rest for a few moments to thicken.

5. Heat a pan or griddle over medium heat and gently coat with coconut oil.

6. Pour 1/4 cup of batter into the griddle for each pancake.

7. Cook for 2-3 minutes, or until bubbles form on the surface and the edges start to set.

8. Flip the pancakes and heat for a further 1-2 minutes or until golden brown and cooked through.

9. Serve warm with your favorite toppings, such as fresh fruit, shredded coconut, or a drizzle of honey or maple syrup.

These breakfast dishes are not only tasty but also quick to make, ensuring you start your day with a fulfilling and healthy meal. Enjoy them as part of your low histamine diet to promote your health and well-being.

CHAPTER FOUR

Simple Lunches Recipe

Salmon Salad

This vivid salad has flaked salmon above a bed of mixed greens, with creamy avocado, juicy cherry tomatoes, and a sprinkling of sesame seeds. Drizzle with olive oil and lemon juice for a pleasant and healthful lunch choice.

Preparation Time: 10 minutes

Cooking Time: 10 minutes (for salmon)

Total Time: 20 minutes

Serving Size: 1

Ingredients:

- 4 ounce salmon fillet
- 2 cups mixed greens
- 1/2 avocado, cut
- 1/2 cup cherry tomatoes, divided
- 1 tablespoon sesame seeds

- Olive oil and lemon juice, for dressing

Method of Preparation:

1. Season salmon fillet with salt and pepper.

2. preheat olive oil in a pan over a moderate flame. Cook salmon for 3-4 minutes on each side, until cooked through.

3. In a large bowl, combine mixed greens with avocado slices and cherry tomatoes.

4. Flake fried fish over the salad.

5. Sprinkle sesame seeds on top.

6. Drizzle with olive oil and lemon juice.

7. Serve immediately and enjoy your healthful salmon salad!

Turkey Lettuce Wraps

These fresh and tasty lettuce wraps are loaded with sliced turkey, creamy avocado, crisp shredded carrots, and cool cucumber sticks. Drizzle with tahini sauce for a tasty and low-carb lunch alternative.

Preparation Time: 10 minutes

Cooking Time: None

Total Time: 10 minutes

Serving Size: 2-3 wraps

Ingredients:

- 6 big lettuce leaves (such as butter or romaine)
- 6 slices turkey breast
- 1/2 avocado, sliced 1/2 cup shredded carrots
- 1/2 cup cucumber sticks
- Tahini sauce, for drizzling

Method of Preparation:

1. Lay out lettuce leaves on a flat surface.

2. Place turkey slices on each lettuce leaf.

3. Top with avocado slices, shredded carrots, and cucumber spears.

4. Drizzle with tahini sauce.

5. Roll up the lettuce leaves like a burrito, enclosing the filling.

6. Secure with toothpicks if required.

7. Serve immediately and enjoy your turkey lettuce wraps!

Quinoa Salad

This vibrant quinoa salad is loaded with flavor and nutrition, with sliced bell peppers, crisp cucumber, sweet cherry tomatoes, salty black olives, and tangy feta cheese. Tossed with tangy olive oil and lemon dressing, it's a filling and healthful lunch alternative.

Preparation Time: 15 minutes

Cooking Time: 15 minutes (for quinoa)

Total Time: 30 minutes

Serving Size: 2

Ingredients:

- 1 cup cooked quinoa
- 1/2 cup chopped bell peppers (assorted hues)
- 1/2 cup diced cucumber
- 1/2 cup cherry tomatoes, halved
- 1/4 cup sliced black olives

- 1/4 cup crumbled feta cheese

- 2 tablespoons minced natural herbs (such as parsley or basil)

- 2 tablespoons olive oil

- 1 tablespoon lemon juice

- Salt & pepper, to taste

Method of Preparation:

1. In a large bowl, add cooked quinoa, diced bell peppers, cucumber, cherry tomatoes, black olives, crumbled feta cheese, and chopped fresh herbs.

2. In a small bowl, mix olive oil, lemon juice, salt, and pepper to create the dressing.

3. Pour the dressing over the quinoa salad and toss until thoroughly incorporated.

4. Taste and adjust seasoning as required.

5. Divide the salad into serving dishes and sprinkle with more fresh herbs if desired.

6. Serve as soon as possible or freeze until ready to eat.

Zucchini Noodles with Pesto

These zucchini noodles, popularly known as zoodles, are tossed in a colorful and savory homemade pesto sauce prepared from fresh basil, pine nuts, garlic, and Parmesan cheese. Top with grilled chicken or tofu for additional protein, or enjoy as a light and refreshing vegetarian alternative.

Preparation Time: 15 minutes

Cooking Time: 10 minutes

Total Time: 25 minutes

Serving Size: 2

Ingredients:

- 2 medium zucchini
- 1/2 cup fresh basil leaves
- 1/4 cup pine nuts
- 1 clove garlic

- 2 tablespoons grated Parmesan cheese

- 2 tablespoons olive oil

- Salt & pepper, to taste

- Grilled chicken or tofu, for serving (optional)

Method of Preparation:

1. Using a spiralizer or vegetable peeler, prepare zucchini noodles (zoodles) from the zucchini.

2. In a food processor or blender, mix fresh basil, pine nuts, garlic, Parmesan cheese, olive oil, salt, and pepper. Blend until smooth and creamy.

3. In a large pan, heat olive oil over a moderate flame. Add zucchini noodles and simmer for 3-4 minutes or until just soft.

4. Add the pesto sauce to the pan with the zucchini noodles and mix until fully covered.

5. Cook for another 1-2 minutes, until heated through.

6. Serve immediately, topped with grilled chicken or tofu if preferred.

Tuna Stuffed Avocado

These creamy avocado halves are stuffed with a tasty blend of canned tuna, crisp celery, tangy red onion, and creamy mayonnaise. Serve as a light and filling lunch option that's filled with protein and healthy fats.

Preparation Time: 10 minutes

Cooking Time: None

Total Time: 10 minutes

Serving Size: 2

Ingredients:

- 2 ripe avocados
- 1 can (5 oz) tuna, drained
- 1/4 cup sliced celery
- 2 tablespoons diced red onion
- 2 tablespoons mayonnaise
- 1 tablespoon lemon juice
- Salt & pepper, to taste

Method of Preparation:

1. Split avocados in half across the middle and eliminate the pits.
2. In a bowl, mix drained tuna, chopped celery, diced red onion, mayonnaise, lemon juice, salt, and pepper.
3. Spoon the tuna mixture into the avocado halves, dividing equally.
4. Serve immediately and enjoy your tuna-packed avocados!

5. These lunch dishes provide a range of tastes and textures, ensuring you have a tasty and healthy midday meal. Whether you favor salads, wraps, or grain-based foods, there's something for everyone to enjoy as part of your low-histamine diet.

CHAPTER FIVE

Flavorful Dinners in Minutes

Chicken with Lemon Herb Grilling

Juicy chicken breasts are grilled to perfection after being marinated in a delectable blend of garlic, olive oil, lemon juice, and fresh herbs. For a nutritious and flavorful supper, serve with steamed veggies of your choice.

Preparation Time: 10 minutes

Cooking Time: 10 minutes

Total Time: 20 minutes

Servings Size: 2

Ingredients

- Two skinless, boneless chicken breasts
- olive oil,
- 2 tablespoons
- 2 minced garlic cloves
- 2 teaspoons lemon juice

- 1 tablespoon chopped fresh herbs (such as rosemary, thyme, or parsley)
- Salt & pepper, to taste

Method of Preparation:

1. In a bowl, mix olive oil, minced garlic, lemon juice, chopped fresh herbs, salt, and pepper to form the marinade.
2. Arrange chicken breasts in a shallow dish and sprinkle the marinade over them, turning to cover evenly.
3. Cover and place in the refrigerator for at least 30 minutes, or as long as four hours.
4. Warm up the grill to medium-high temperature. Remove chicken from marinade and discard excess marinade.
5. Grill chicken for 6-8 minutes on each side, or until cooked through and juices run clear.

6. Remove off grill and allow to rest for a few minutes before serving.

7. Serve grilled lemon herb chicken with steamed veggies or your favorite side dishes.

Baked Salmon with Asparagus

This easy and beautiful recipe combines delicate salmon fillets seasoned with salt, pepper, and lemon zest, and baked with fresh asparagus stalks till perfectly cooked. Serve with a squeeze of fresh lemon juice for a punch of flavor.

Preparation Time: 10 minutes

Cooking Time: 10 minutes

Total Time: 20 minutes

Serving Size: 2

Ingredients

- 2 salmon fillets
- 1 bunch asparagus, trimmed
- olive oil, 2 tablespoons

- 1 tablespoon lemon zest

- Salt & pepper, to taste

- Lemon wedges, for serving

Method of Preparation:

1. Warm up oven to 400°F (200°C). Wrap a baking sheet with paper parchment.

2. Place salmon fillets on one side of the baking sheet and lay trimmed asparagus stalks on the other side.

3. Drizzle olive oil over the fish and asparagus. Sprinkle lemon zest, salt, and pepper over both.

4. Toss asparagus to coat evenly with oil and spice.

5. Bake for 12-15 minutes, or until salmon is cooked through and flakes readily with a fork.

6. Remove from oven and allow to rest for a few minutes.

7. Serve cooked salmon and asparagus with lemon wedges for squeezing over the top.

Stir-fried shrimp with Vegetables

Succulent shrimp are stir-fried with a colorful array of veggies, including bell peppers, snap peas, and broccoli, in a tasty sauce prepared from tamari, ginger, and garlic. Serve overcooked rice or quinoa for a pleasant and healthful supper.

Preparation Time: 15 minutes

Cooking Time: 10 minutes

Total Time: 25 minutes

Serving Size: 2

Ingredients

- 8 ounces shrimp, peeled and deveined
- 1 cup mixed bell peppers, sliced
- 1 cup snap peas
- 1 cup broccoli florets

- 2 crushed garlic cloves

- 1 tablespoon grated ginger

- 2 tablespoons tamari or soy sauce

- 1 tablespoon sesame oil

- Cooked rice or quinoa, for serving

- Sesame seeds, for garnish

Method of Preparation:

1. Warm the sesame oil in a big pan or wok over medium-high heat.

2. Add minced garlic and grated ginger to the pan and sauté for 1 minute, until fragrant.

3. Add shrimp to the skillet and cook for 2-3 minutes each side, until pink and cooked through. Remove shrimp from pan and put aside.

4. Add sliced bell peppers, snap peas, and broccoli florets to the skillet. Stir-fry for 3-4 minutes until veggies are crisp-tender.

5. Return cooked shrimp to the pan and add tamari or soy sauce. Stir to mix and coat everything evenly.

6. Cook for another 1-2 minutes, until heated through.

7. Serve stir-fried shrimp and veggies over cooked rice or quinoa.

8. Garnish with sesame seeds before serving.

Eggplant Rollatini

Thin slices of grilled eggplant are stuffed with a delicious combination of ricotta cheese, spinach, and herbs, then wrapped up and baked with marinara sauce till bubbling and golden. Serve as a vegetarian main meal that's both stylish and fulfilling.

Preparation Time: 20 minutes

Cooking Time: 30 minutes

Total Time: 50 minutes

Serving Size: 2-3

Ingredients:

- 1 big eggplant, cut lengthwise into thin strips
- 1 cup ricotta cheese
- 1 cup chopped spinach
- 1/4 cup grated Parmesan cheese
- 1 egg, beaten

- 1 clove garlic, minced

- 1 tablespoon chopped fresh basil

- 1 tablespoon chopped fresh parsley

- 1 cup marinara sauce

- Salt & pepper, to taste

Method of Preparation:

1. Warm grill or grill pan at medium to high heat.

2. Brush eggplant slices with olive oil and season with salt and pepper.

3. Grilled eggplant pieces for 2-3 minutes on each side, until soft and grill marks form. Remove from grill and put aside.

4. In a bowl, add ricotta cheese, chopped spinach, grated Parmesan cheese, beaten egg, minced garlic, chopped fresh basil, and chopped fresh parsley. Season with salt and pepper to taste.

5. Spread a dollop of marinara sauce in the bottom of a baking dish.

6. Place a dollop of the ricotta mixture on each grilled eggplant slice and fold it firmly.

7. Place rolled eggplant slices seam-side down in the baking dish.

8. Spoon leftover marinara sauce over the top of the eggplant rollatini.

9. Bake in preheated oven for 20-25 minutes, until bubbling and brown.

10. Serve hot, topped with more chopped fresh herbs as preferred.

Turkey Meatballs on Zucchini Noodles:

These soft turkey meatballs are seasoned with garlic and Italian flavor, then baked till golden brown and cooked through. Serve over spiralized zucchini noodles with marinara sauce for a low-carb and tasty meal alternative.

Preparation Time: 15 minutes

Cooking Time: 25 minutes

Total Time: 40 minutes

Serving Size: 2-3

Ingredients:

- 1 pound ground turkey
- 1/4 cup breadcrumbs (or almond flour for gluten-free)
- 1 egg
- 2 minced garlic cloves
- 1 teaspoon Italian seasoning
- Salt & pepper, to taste

- 2 zucchini, spiralized into noodles

- 1 cup marinara sauce

- Fresh parsley, for garnish

Method of Preparation:

1. Preheat oven to 400°F (200°C). Line a baking sheet with parchment paper.

2. In a large bowl, mix ground turkey, breadcrumbs, egg, chopped garlic, Italian seasoning, salt, and pepper. Mix until completely blended.

3. Shape the mixture into meatballs and put them on the prepared baking sheet.

4. Broil meatball in the hot oven for 20 to 25 minutes, till golden brown and fried through.

5. While the meatballs are baking, prepare the marinara sauce in a pan over medium heat.

6. Add spiralized zucchini noodles to the pan and stir with the marinara sauce until cooked through.

7. Once the meatballs are done, remove them from the oven and arrange them on top of the zucchini noodles.

8. Garnish with fresh parsley before serving.

These evening dishes provide a range of tastes and textures, ensuring you have a full and healthy meal to conclude your day. Whether you favor grilled meats, seafood meals, or vegetarian alternatives, there's something for everyone to enjoy as part of your low-histamine diet.

CHAPTER SIX

Smoothies To Revitalize Your Senses

Green Detox Smoothie:

This colorful green smoothie is filled with detoxifying vegetables including spinach, kale, and cucumber, along with crisp green apple and zesty lemon. Coconut water increases hydration, making it the ideal morning pick-me-up or post-workout refreshment.

Preparation Time: 5 minutes

Total Time: 5 minutes

Serving Size: 1

Ingredients:

- 1 cup spinach leaves
- 1 cup kale leaves, stems
- 1/2 cucumber, peeled and cut
- 1 green apple, cored and cut
- Juice of 1/2 lemon

- 1 cup coconut water

- Optional: ice cubes

Method of Preparation:

1. Place all items in a blender.

2. Blend until smooth and creamy.

3. If preferred, add ice cubes for a cooler smoothie.

4. Pour into a glass and drink immediately.

Tropical Mango Smoothie:

This delightful smoothie brings you to the tropics with its sweet and tangy taste mix of mango, pineapple, and coconut. Greek yogurt adds creaminess and protein, making it a pleasant and healthful breakfast or snack alternative.

Preparation Time: 5 minutes

Total Time: 5 minutes

Serving Size: 1

Ingredients:

- 1 cup frozen mango chunks
- 1/2 cup frozen pineapple chunks
- 1/2 cup Greek yogurt
- 1/2 cup coconut milk
- Juice of 1/2 lime
- Optional: honey or maple syrup, to taste

Method of Preparation:

1. Place all items in a blender.
2. Blend until smooth and creamy.
3. Taste and make changes in sweetness if needed through the addition of honey or maple syrup to it.
4. Pour into a glass and drink immediately.

Berry Blast Smoothie:

This antioxidant-rich smoothie has a combination of mixed berries, including strawberries, blueberries, and raspberries, blended with banana, spinach, and almond milk for a healthy and delightful start to your day.

Preparation Time: 5 minutes

Total Time: 5 minutes

Serving Size: 1

Ingredients:

- 1/2 cup frozen mixed berries (strawberries, blueberries, raspberries)
- 1/2 ripe banana, frozen
- 1 cup spinach leaves
- 1/2 cup almond milk
- Optional: 1 tablespoon chia seeds or flaxseeds
- Optional: honey or maple syrup, to taste

Method of Preparation:

1. Place all items in a blender.

2. Blend until smooth and creamy.

3. If preferred, add chia seeds or flaxseeds for extra fiber and omega-3s.

4. Taste and modify the sugar if required by adding honey or maple syrup as needed.

5. Pour into a glass and drink immediately.

Chocolate Peanut Butter Smoothie:

Indulge your sweet craving with this luscious smoothie that tastes like a milkshake but is filled with healthful ingredients like cocoa powder, peanut butter, banana, and spinach. It's the ultimate guilt-free treat for any time of day.

Preparation Time: 5 minutes

Total Time: 5 minutes

Serving Size: 1

Ingredients:

- 1 ripe banana, frozen
- 1 tablespoon cocoa powder
- 1 tbsp peanut butter
- 1 cup spinach leaves
- 1 cup almond milk
- Optional: honey or maple syrup, to taste

Method of Preparation:

1. Place all items in a blender.
2. Blend until smooth and creamy.
3. Try varying the sweetness if wished for by adding honey or maple syrup as needed.
4. Pour into a glass and drink immediately.

Pineapple Coconut Smoothie:

This tropical-inspired smoothie mixes sweet and juicy pineapple with creamy coconut milk and Greek yogurt for a pleasant and fulfilling beverage. Shredded coconut adds texture and taste, making it seem like a small vacation in a glass.

Preparation Time: 5 minutes

Total Time: 5 minutes

Serving Size: 1

Ingredients:

- 1 cup frozen pineapple chunks
- 1/2 cup coconut milk
- 1/2 cup Greek yogurt
- 2 teaspoons shredded coconut
- Optional: honey or maple syrup, to taste

Method of Preparation:

1. Place all items in a blender.

2. Blend until smooth and creamy.

3. Try varying sweetness if needed by combining honey or maple syrup.

4. Pour into a glass and drink immediately.

5. These smoothie recipes are not only tasty but also healthy, giving a quick way to pack in vitamins, minerals, and antioxidants to power your day.

6. Whether you like green detox smoothies, fruity blends, or rich chocolate delights, there's a smoothie choice for every taste preference and nutritional necessity.

CHAPTER SEVEN

Side Dishes and Salads

Garlic Roasted Brussels Sprouts

These crisp Brussels sprouts are roasted to perfection with garlic, olive oil, and a sprinkling of Parmesan cheese, resulting in a savory and enticing side dish that matches well with any main meal.

Preparation Time: 10 minutes

Cooking Time: 25 minutes

Total Time: 35 minutes

Serving Size: 2-4

Ingredients:

- 1 pound Brussels sprouts, trimmed and halved
- 2 tablespoons olive oil
- 2 cloves garlic, minced

- Salt & pepper, to taste

- 2 tablespoons grated Parmesan cheese

Method of Preparation

1. Preheat oven to 400°F (200°C). Line a baking sheet with parchment paper.

2. In a large bowl, mix Brussels sprouts with olive oil, minced garlic, salt, and pepper until equally coated.

3. Spread Brussels sprouts in a single layer on the prepared baking sheet.

4. Roast in preheated oven for 20-25 minutes, stirring halfway through, until golden brown and tender.

5. Sprinkle roasted Brussels sprouts with grated Parmesan cheese before serving.

Quinoa and Vegetable Stir-Fry

This colorful stir-fry combines fluffy quinoa with a variety of sautéed veggies, including bell peppers, carrots, snap peas, and broccoli, in a flavorful soy ginger sauce. Serve as a healthful and nutritious side dish or light vegetarian main entrée.

Preparation Time: 15 minutes

Cooking Time: 15 minutes

Total Time: 30 minutes

Serving Size: 4

Ingredients:

- 1 cup quinoa, washed
- 2 cups water or vegetable broth
- 2 tablespoons olive oil
- 2 cloves garlic, minced
- 1 tablespoon grated ginger
- 1 bell pepper, sliced 1 carrot, julienned

- 1 cup snap peas

- 1 cup broccoli florets

- 2 tablespoons soy sauce or tamari

- 1 tablespoon rice vinegar

- 1 teaspoon sesame oil

- Optional: If possible the seeds of sesame and cut green onions, for garnishes

Method of Preparation

1. In a medium saucepan, mix quinoa and water or vegetable broth. Bring to a boil, then decrease heat, cover, and simmer for 15-20 minutes, or until quinoa is cooked and liquid is absorbed.

2. In a big pan or skillet, warm olive oil over moderately high heat. Add minced garlic and grated ginger, and simmer for 1 minute, until fragrant.

3. Add sliced bell pepper, julienned carrot, snap peas, and broccoli florets to the skillet. Stir-fry for 5-6 minutes, or until veggies are crisp-tender.

4. In a small bowl, mix soy sauce or tamari, rice vinegar, and sesame oil to produce the sauce.

5. Add cooked quinoa to the pan with the stir-fried veggies. Pour the sauce over the quinoa and veggies, and toss until everything is completely covered.

6. Cook for another 2-3 minutes, until heated through.

7. Serve quinoa and vegetable stir-fry hot, topped with sesame seeds and sliced green onions if preferred.

Roasted Sweet Potatoes with Herbs

These roasted sweet potatoes are seasoned with a combination of fresh herbs, garlic, and olive oil, resulting in a tasty and fragrant side dish that's both sweet and salty. Serve as a healthful addition to any meal.

Preparation Time: 10 minutes

Cooking Time: 30 minutes

Total Time: 40 minutes

Serving Size: 2-4

Ingredients:

- 2 big sweet potatoes, peeled and cubed
- 2 tablespoons olive oil
- 2 cloves garlic, minced
- 1 tablespoon chopped fresh rosemary
- 1 tablespoon chopped fresh thyme
- Salt & pepper, to taste

Method of Preparation

1. Preheat oven to 400°F (200°C). Line a baking sheet with parchment paper.

2. In a large bowl, combine sweet potato cubes with olive oil, minced garlic, chopped fresh rosemary, chopped fresh thyme, salt, and pepper until equally coated.

3. Spread sweet potato cubes in a single layer on the prepared baking sheet.

4. Roast in preheated oven for 25-30 minutes, stirring halfway through, until golden brown and tender.

5. Serve roasted sweet potatoes with herbs hot as a delightful side dish.

Sauteed Garlic Spinach

This fast and simple side dish comprises crisp baby spinach leaves sautéed with garlic and olive oil till wilted and delicious. Serve as a healthful complement to any meal, giving a splash of brilliant green color to your dish.

Preparation Time: 5 minutes

Cooking Time: 5 minutes

Total Time: 10 minutes

Serving Size: 2-4

Ingredients

- 8 ounces baby spinach leaves
- 2 tablespoons olive oil
- 2 cloves garlic, minced
- Salt & pepper, to taste

Method of Preparation

- Warm olive oil in a big pan over a moderate flame.

- Add minced garlic to the pan and sauté for 1 minute, until fragrant.

- Add baby spinach leaves to the pan in batches, stirring with tongs until wilted.

- Continue cooking until all spinach leaves are wilted and soft, approximately 2-3 minutes.

- Season sautéed garlic spinach with salt and pepper to taste.

- Serve hot as a delightful and healthful side dish.

Cauliflower Rice Pilaf

This light and tasty cauliflower rice pilaf is produced by sautéing cauliflower rice with onions, garlic, and a combination of fragrant spices. Finished with fresh parsley and toasted almonds, it's a tasty and low-carb alternative to typical rice pilaf.

Preparation Time: 10 minutes

Cooking Time: 15 minutes

Total Time: 25 minutes

Serving Size: 4

Ingredients:

- 1 medium head cauliflower, riced
- 2 tablespoons olive oil
- 1 onion, finely chopped
- 2 cloves garlic, minced
- 1 teaspoon ground cumin
- 1/2 teaspoon ground turmeric

- 1/2 teaspoon ground coriander
- Salt & pepper, to taste
- 1/4 cup chopped fresh parsley
- 1/4 cup sliced almonds, toasted

Method of Preparation

1. Cut cauliflower into florets and pulse in a food processor until it resembles rice.
2. Warm olive oil in a big pan over a medium-high flame.
3. Add finely chopped onion to the pan and sauté for 3-4 minutes, until softened.
4. Add minced garlic to the pan and sauté for 1 minute, until fragrant.
5. Stir in cauliflower rice, ground cumin, ground turmeric, and ground coriander. Sprinkle with a little pepper and salt according to your preference.

6. Cook, stirring periodically, for 8-10 minutes, until cauliflower rice is soft and heated through.

7. Remove from heat and mix in chopped fresh parsley and toasted sliced almonds.

8. Serve cauliflower rice pilaf hot as a delightful and healthful side dish.

CHAPTER EIGHT

Tips for Shopping and Meal Planning

Choose Fresh Meals: Opt for fresh, unprocessed meals wherever feasible. Shop for fresh meats, poultry, fish, fruits, and vegetables to decrease histamine consumption.

Read Labels Carefully: When buying packaged or processed foods, carefully read ingredient labels to avoid goods containing histamine-rich substances or additions.

Plan Meals: Take time to plan your meals and snacks to ensure they correspond with a low histamine diet. This might help you avoid last-minute temptations or convenience items that may not be acceptable.

Rotate Foods: Rotate your dietary selections to prevent overdosing on any one sort of food.

Variety is crucial to having a balanced and healthy diet while avoiding histamine exposure.

Consider Food Preparation Techniques: Opt for cooking techniques that decrease histamine generation, such as boiling, steaming, or grilling fresh foods. Avoid cooking procedures that include age or fermentation, such as curing or smoking.

Be Mindful of Cross-Contamination: Take steps to avoid cross-contamination between histamine-rich foods and fresh foods during preparation and storage. Use separate cutting boards, cutlery, and storage containers for histamine-containing foods.

14-Day Low Histamine Diet Meal Plan:

Day 1:

Breakfast: Blueberry Banana Smoothie

Lunch: Salmon Salad

Dinner: Chicken with Lemon Herb Grilling

Snack: Sauteed Garlic Spinach

Day 2:

Breakfast: Quinoa Breakfast Bowl

Lunch: Turkey Lettuce Wraps

Dinner: Baked Salmon with Asparagus

Snack: Berry Blast Smoothie

Day 3:

Breakfast: Chia Seed Pudding

Lunch: Quinoa Salad

Dinner: Stir-Fried Shrimp with Vegetables

Snack: Roasted Sweet Potatoes with Herbs

Day 4:

Breakfast: Egg Muffins

Lunch: Zucchini Noodles with Pesto

Dinner: Eggplant Rollatini

Snack: Chocolate Peanut Butter Smoothie

Day 5:

Breakfast: Coconut Flour Pancakes

Lunch: Tuna Stuffed Avocado

Dinner: Turkey Meatballs on Zucchini Noodles

Snack: Pineapple Coconut Smoothie

Day 6:

Breakfast: Green Detox Smoothie

Lunch: Salmon Salad

Dinner: Chicken with Lemon Herb Grilling

Snack: Garlic Roasted Brussels Sprouts

Day 7:

Breakfast: Tropical Mango Smoothie

Lunch: Turkey Lettuce Wraps

Dinner: Baked Salmon with Asparagus

Snack: Quinoa and Vegetable Stir-Fry

Day 8:

Breakfast: Blueberry Banana Smoothie

Lunch: Quinoa Salad

Dinner: Stir-Fried Shrimp with Vegetables

Snack: Sauteed Garlic Spinach

Day 9:

Breakfast: Quinoa Breakfast Bowl

Lunch: Zucchini Noodles with Pesto

Dinner: Eggplant Rollatini

Snack: Berry Blast Smoothie

Day 10:

Breakfast: Chia Seed Pudding

Lunch: Tuna Stuffed Avocado

Dinner: Turkey Meatballs on Zucchini Noodles

Snack: Chocolate Peanut Butter Smoothie

Day 11:

Breakfast: Coconut Flour Pancakes

Lunch: Salmon Salad

Dinner: Chicken with Lemon Herb Grilling

Snack: Pineapple Coconut Smoothie

Day 12:

Breakfast: Green Detox Smoothie

Lunch: Turkey Lettuce Wraps

Dinner: Baked Salmon with Asparagus

Snack: Garlic Roasted Brussels Sprouts

Day 13:

Breakfast: Tropical Mango Smoothie

Lunch: Quinoa Salad

Dinner: Stir-Fried Shrimp with Vegetables

Snack: Quinoa and Vegetable Stir-Fry

Day 14:

Breakfast: Blueberry Banana Smoothie

Lunch: Zucchini Noodles with Pesto

Dinner: Eggplant Rollatini

Snack: Sauteed Garlic Spinach

This 14-day meal plan incorporates a variety of delicious and nutritious recipes suitable for a low histamine diet. Adjust portion sizes and snacks according to individual dietary needs and preferences.

CHAPTER NINE

Special Occasion Feasts

Celebratory Recipes for Holidays and Gatherings

Hosting parties and celebrating holidays can be pleasant times filled with excellent food and treasured memories. However, for persons with histamine sensitivity, managing these events might bring particular obstacles. Fear not! This part of the cookbook is devoted to providing you with a repertoire of festive meals that suit your dietary demands without sacrificing flavor or tradition.

Hosting Guests with Histamine Intolerance

When entertaining visitors with histamine intolerance, it's crucial to establish a friendly and inclusive setting so everyone can enjoy the celebrations. Consider sending out invites with a quick message regarding your understanding of their dietary restrictions and reassure them that you've made efforts to suit their requirements. Here are some recommendations for welcoming visitors with histamine intolerance:

Communication is Key: Reach out to your visitors ahead of time to learn about their unique dietary limitations and preferences. This will help you to arrange your menu correctly and guarantee that there are plenty of selections accessible for everyone.

Offer a Variety of alternatives: Prepare a broad assortment of foods that appeal to various dietary demands, including low histamine alternatives. This might include fresh salads, grilled meats, veggie side dishes, and gluten-free or dairy-free options.

Label Your Dishes: Clearly label each dish with its components to enable visitors with histamine sensitivity to locate safe alternatives. You may use basic labels like "low histamine," "gluten-free," or "dairy-free" to make it easy for everyone to navigate the buffet.

Be Mindful of Cross-Contamination: Take steps to prevent cross-contamination between dishes to avoid mistakenly exposing visitors to allergies or high-histamine substances. Use separate utensils, cutting boards, and serving platters for various foods, and consider offering individual servings for visitors with severe allergies.

Empower Your Visitors: Encourage visitors with histamine intolerance to bring their dishes or ingredients if they're worried about the menu. This will offer them a piece of mind knowing that they have safe alternatives accessible, and it demonstrates that you appreciate their dietary demands.

Tips for Modifying Traditional Favorites

Transforming classic Christmas treats into low-histamine alternatives doesn't mean compromising taste or tradition. With a little imagination and innovation, you may reproduce classic recipes that everyone will appreciate. Here are some recommendations for tweaking classic favorites:

Focus on Fresh items: Opt for fresh, seasonal items wherever feasible, since they tend to have lower histamine levels than processed or aged meals. Choose fruits and vegetables that are in season, and emphasize organic alternatives to avoid exposure to pesticides and chemicals.

Experiment with Flavorful Substitutes: Explore alternative ingredients and taste profiles to add depth and variety to your cuisine. For example, you may add fresh herbs, spices, citrus zest, and aromatic vegetables like onions and garlic to improve the flavor of your meals without depending on high-histamine items.

Get Creative with Cooking Techniques: Experiment with various cooking techniques, such as grilling, roasting, steaming, and sautéing, to bring out the natural tastes of your food. These strategies may help retain the nutritional integrity of your food while decreasing the development of histamines.

Consider Texture and Appearance: Pay attention to the texture and appearance of your foods to make them visually attractive and pleasurable to consume. Incorporate a range of textures, such as crispy, crunchy, creamy, and chewy, to create a more dynamic eating experience.

Don't Forget About Dessert: No Christmas feast is complete without a sweet treat! Get creative with low-histamine dessert alternatives like fruit sorbets, coconut milk-based ice creams, or allergen-friendly baked goodies.

Experiment with other sweeteners like honey, maple syrup, or stevia to fulfill your sweet taste without causing histamine sensitivity.

By following these suggestions and recipes, you may arrange unforgettable celebrations and gatherings that accommodate the nutritional requirements of all your visitors, including those with histamine intolerance. With a little forethought and imagination, you can enjoy excellent cuisine and make memorable memories together.

CHAPTER TEN

Beyond the Plate: Lifestyle Tips

In our path towards greater health and well-being, food choices are just one piece of the jigsaw. This portion of the cookbook goes into holistic lifestyle ideas that complement your low-histamine diet, allowing you to enhance your overall health and energy.

Managing Stress and Sleep for Better Health

Stress and poor sleep may substantially damage our physical and mental well-being, aggravating symptoms of histamine intolerance and undermining our attempts to maintain a healthy lifestyle. Here are some ways to control stress and enhance sleep quality:

Practice Stress Reduction Tactics: Incorporate stress reduction tactics into your everyday routine to promote relaxation and peace.

This might involve mindfulness meditation, deep breathing techniques, yoga, tai chi, or progressive muscular relaxation. Find activities that connect with you and make them a regular component of your self-care regimen.

Prioritize Sleep Hygiene: Create a suitable sleep environment that promotes comfortable and restorative sleep. Establish a regular sleep routine by going to bed and getting up at the same time every day, including on weekends. Keep your bedroom dark, quiet, and cool, and invest in a comfortable mattress and pillows to assist healthy sleep. Limit exposure to screens and stimulating activities before sleep, and avoid coffee and large meals close to bedtime.

Mindful Eating Practices: Pay attention to your eating patterns and how they may be impacted by stress or emotional triggers. Practice mindful eating by enjoying each mouthful, chewing carefully, and tuning into your body's hunger and fullness signals. Cultivate a healthy connection with food by approaching mealtimes with appreciation and mindfulness, rather than as a source of stress or worry.

Engage in calming Activities: Incorporate calming activities into your everyday routine to help unwind and de-stress. This may involve taking a warm bath, listening to relaxing music, reading a book, spending time in nature, or indulging in creative activities like painting, gardening, or writing. Find hobbies that offer you pleasure and relaxation, and make time for them frequently to replenish your batteries.

Incorporating Movement and Exercise

Regular physical exercise is vital for maintaining overall health and well-being, supporting appropriate digestion, circulation, and immunological function. Here are some strategies for adding movement and exercise into your everyday routine:

Find Activities You Enjoy: Choose things that you like and look forward to, whether it's walking, running, swimming, dancing, cycling, or practicing yoga. Incorporate a range of activities to keep things interesting and avoid boredom.

Start softly and Build Consistency: If you're new to exercising or have been inactive for a long, start softly and gradually increase the intensity and length of your exercises over time.

Aim for at least 30 minutes of moderate-intensity exercise most days of the week, and find chances to move throughout the day, such as taking the stairs instead of the elevator or going for a brief stroll during your lunch break.

Listen to Your Body: Pay attention to how your body reacts to exercise and alter your regimen appropriately. If you encounter pain or discomfort, take a break and allow your body time to relax and recuperate. Be cognizant of any limits or constraints caused by your histamine intolerance, and select activities that are gentle on your body while yet offering decent exercise.

Stay Flexible and adaptable: Be flexible and adaptable with your workout program, particularly if you're struggling with variable energy levels or symptoms of histamine intolerance. Modify your exercises as required to suit any changes in your health or circumstances, and don't be hesitant to attempt new activities or explore other fitness techniques that correspond with your requirements and interests.

Strategies for Dining Out and Traveling

Navigating restaurants and travel may offer unique obstacles for persons with histamine intolerance, but with good planning and preparation, you can still enjoy eating out and visiting new areas. Here are some methods for eating out and traveling with histamine intolerance:

investigate Restaurants Ahead of Time: Before eating out, investigate restaurants in your region that provide low histamine alternatives or can accommodate particular dietary demands. Look for menus that emphasize fresh, healthy foods and avoid meals that are likely to include high-histamine items like aged cheeses, cured meats, and fermented foods.

Convey your preferences: When booking a reservation or ordering at a restaurant, don't hesitate to convey your dietary preferences clearly and respectfully to the staff. Ask inquiries regarding ingredients and cooking techniques, and seek tweaks or replacements as required to make your dish low histamine-friendly.

Be Prepared with Snacks: When traveling, carry a supply of low-histamine snacks and portable meal alternatives to keep you fuelled and satisfied on the move. This might include fresh fruit, raw veggies, nuts and seeds, rice cakes, hummus, and homemade energy snacks. Having snacks on hand can help avoid hunger-induced food cravings and make it simpler to adhere to your dietary plan when traveling.

Choose Accommodating lodgings: When reserving lodgings for your vacation, seek alternatives that include cooking facilities or give access to a refrigerator and microwave. This will enable you to cook basic meals and snacks in your hotel and keep perishable products properly, decreasing your dependency on eating out for every meal.

Pack Your Essentials: Bring along any nutritional supplements or medicines you may need to treat your histamine sensitivity while traveling. This might include antihistamines, digestive enzymes, probiotics, or any other nutrients advised by your healthcare professional. Make sure to bring them in your carry-on baggage to ensure they're conveniently accessible throughout your vacation.

keep Hydrated and Well-Rested: Drink lots of water and keep hydrated when traveling to support your body's natural detoxification processes and decrease the risk of dehydration, which may increase symptoms of histamine intolerance. Aim to get enough rest and prioritize sleep, particularly if you're moving time zones or transitioning to a new schedule.

By adopting these lifestyle guidelines into your daily routine, you may enhance your overall health and well-being while controlling histamine sensitivity via food and lifestyle alterations. Remember to listen to your body, prioritize self-care, and seek help from healthcare experts and loved ones as required on your road to improved health.

CONCLUSION

As we approach the conclusion of our culinary adventure into the world of low histamine eating, it's crucial to reflect on the major takeaways, congratulate your successes, and explore ways to stay connected with the community for continuing support and inspiration.

Recap of Key Takeaways

Throughout this cookbook, we've dug into the subtleties of histamine intolerance and how dietary choices may play a significant part in controlling symptoms and increasing overall well-being. Here's a review of some essential lessons to remember:

Understanding Histamine Intolerance: Educate yourself on histamine intolerance, its symptoms, and typical triggers to make educated food choices that support your health.

The Basics of a Low Histamine Diet: Embrace the concepts of a low histamine diet, concentrating on fresh, whole foods while avoiding high-histamine products and processed meals.

fast and simple dishes: Discover a varied assortment of fast and simple dishes that adapt to your dietary demands without compromising flavor or convenience.

Lifestyle Tips: Incorporate holistic lifestyle habits such as stress management, regular exercise, and mindful eating to promote your general health and well-being.

Strategies for Dining Out and Traveling: Learn how to navigate restaurants and travel with confidence, equipped with information and practical ideas for remaining on track with your low histamine diet.

Encouragement for Continued Success

Embarking on a road towards greater health and well-being is a respectable undertaking, and your dedication to controlling histamine intolerance via food and lifestyle alterations is incredibly inspirational. As you continue on this journey, remember to:

Be Patient and Persistent: Managing histamine intolerance is a journey, not a destination. Be patient with yourself as you manage dietary modifications and lifestyle adjustments, and don't be discouraged by setbacks or hurdles along the road. Stay focused on your objectives and appreciate your accomplishments, no matter how modest.

Listen to Your Body: Pay attention to how various meals and lifestyle variables impact your body and symptoms of histamine intolerance. Trust your instincts and listen to your body's messages, making changes as required to maintain your health and well-being.

Seek Support and Resources: You're not alone on this road. Reach out to healthcare experts, support groups, and online forums for assistance, encouragement, and friendship. Share your stories, ask questions, and provide support to those experiencing similar issues.

Celebrate Your achievements: Celebrate your achievements and milestones along the road, no matter how tiny. Whether it's attempting a new low histamine dish, adhering to your food plan during a social event, or detecting changes in your symptoms, take time to identify and celebrate your successes.

How to Stay Connected with the Community

Staying connected with the community is crucial for continued support, inspiration, and companionship on your path toward greater health. Here are several methods to keep connected:

Join Online Communities: Participate in online forums, social media groups, and support networks devoted to histamine intolerance and low histamine lifestyle. Connect with people who have similar experiences, ask questions, and exchange information and insights.

Attend Support Groups: Seek out local support groups or meetings for folks with histamine intolerance. Meeting people face-to-face may give you a feeling of camaraderie and support, and you may acquire useful ideas and methods from others in your community.

Follow Blogs and Websites: Stay informed and motivated by following blogs, websites, and social media accounts devoted to histamine intolerance, low histamine recipes, and holistic health. Subscribe to newsletters, podcasts, and other resources to remain up-to-date on the newest research and advances in the area.

Engage with Authors and specialists: Connect with authors, chefs, nutritionists, and other specialists on the subject of histamine intolerance and low histamine living. Attend seminars, webinars, and events, and reach out to authors and experts for information, direction, and support.

By remaining connected with the community, you may gain strength, inspiration, and encouragement from others on similar journeys and establish a supporting network of allies who understand and sympathize with your experiences. Together, we may continue to learn, develop, and flourish on our road toward improved health and well-being.

www.ingramcontent.com/pod-product-compliance
Lightning Source LLC
Chambersburg PA
CBHW070814260726
48660CB00005B/1847